Five Little Kittens

Written by Jody Silver

Illustrated by A. J. MacGregor

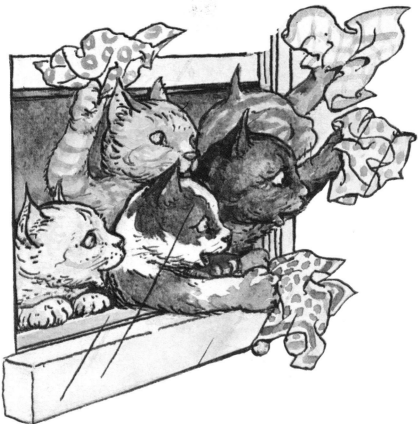

Happytime Books

Dutton-Elsevier Publishing Company, Inc.

New York

Mama Cat fluffed and brushed and combed and fussed over herself before going out shopping. "Be perfect dears, no mischief, no tears," she said. "And I'll bring each of you back something special.

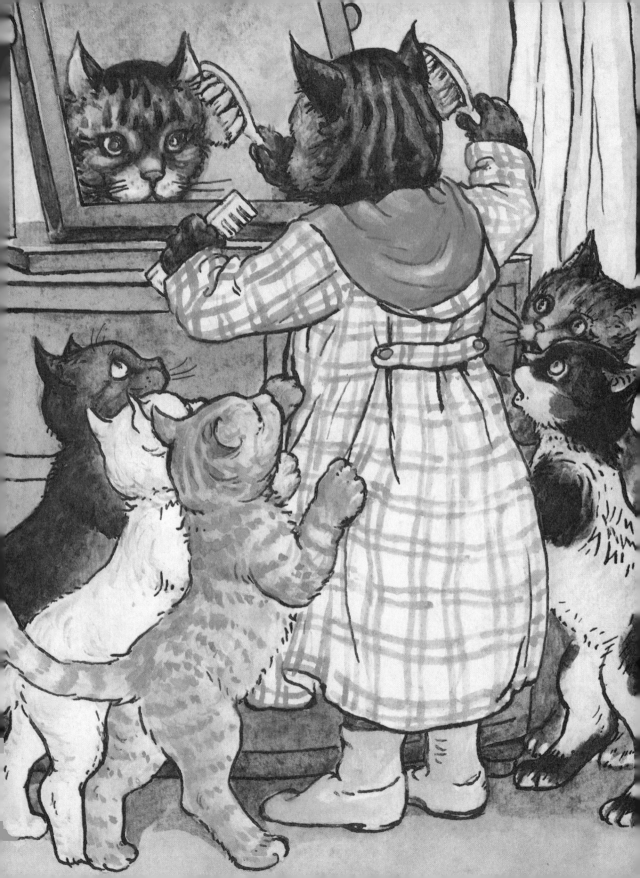

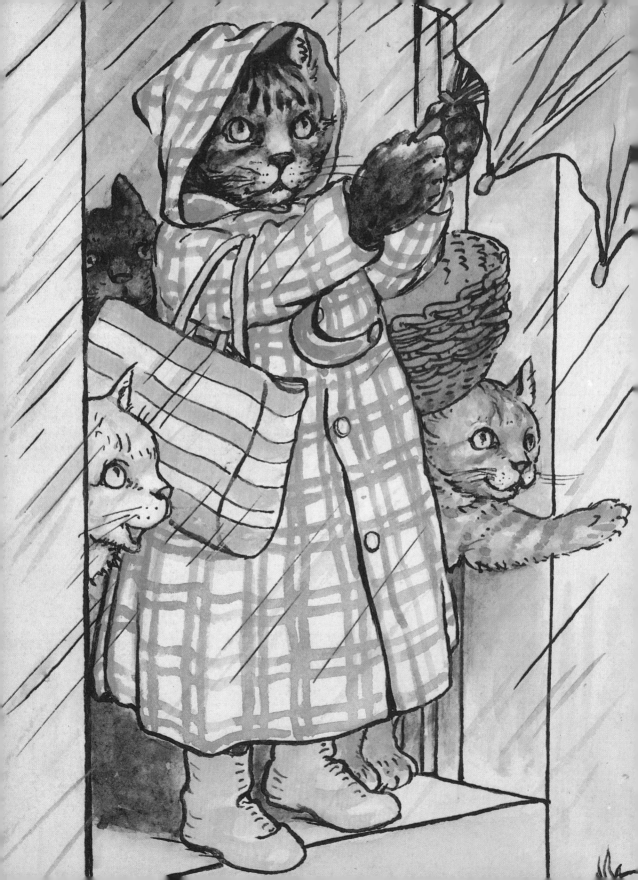

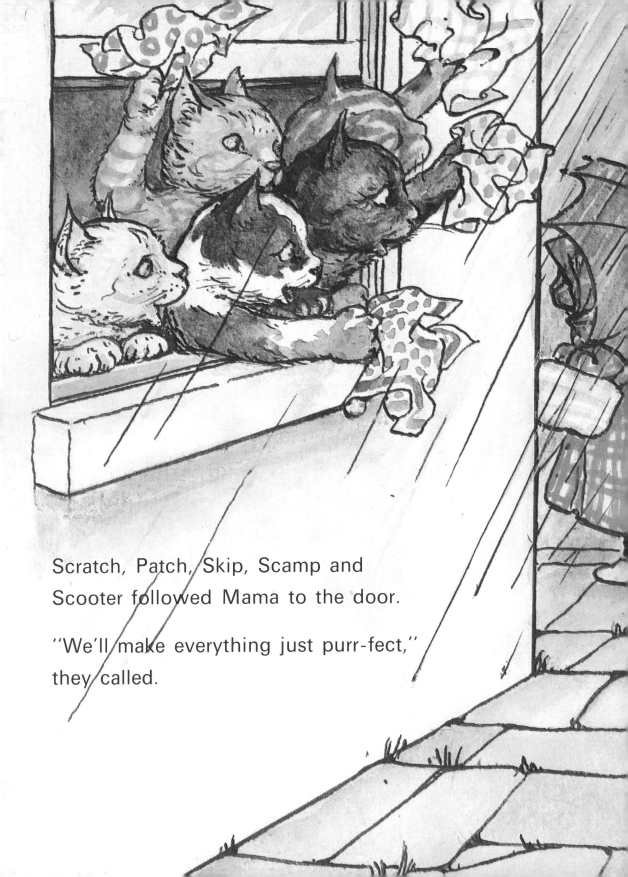

Scratch, Patch, Skip, Scamp and
Scooter followed Mama to the door.

"We'll make everything just purr-fect,"
they called.

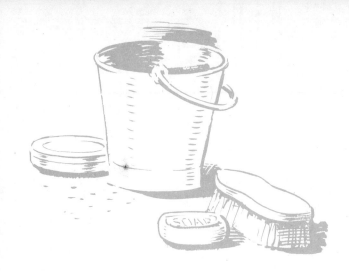

It was Scratch who said she'd scrub
the pots and pans and wash the tub.
She put on Mama's apron to keep from
getting wet.

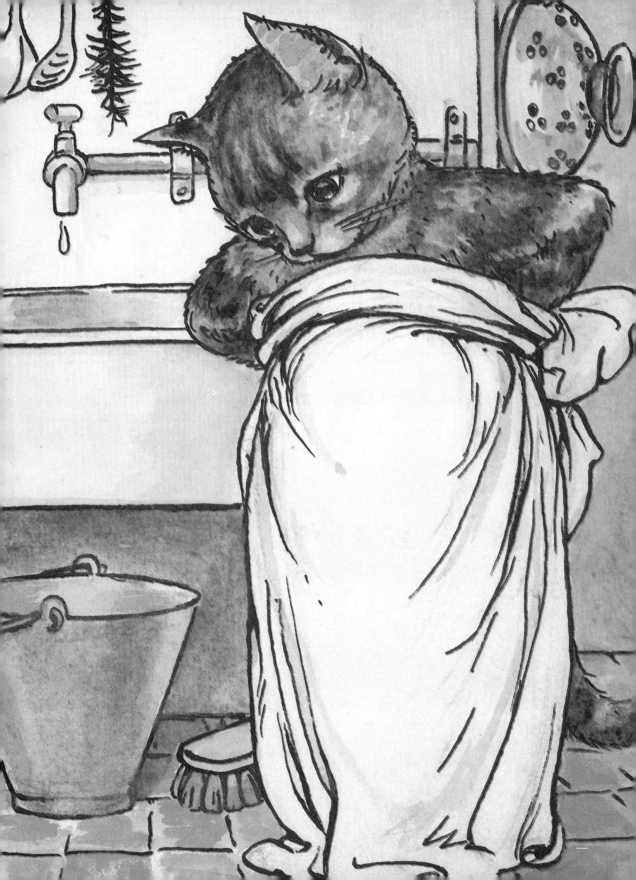

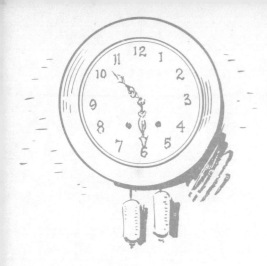

Patch grabbed the brush and dustpan,
Scooter got the broom.
Skip went to clean up breakfast,
Scamp said, "I'll do my room."

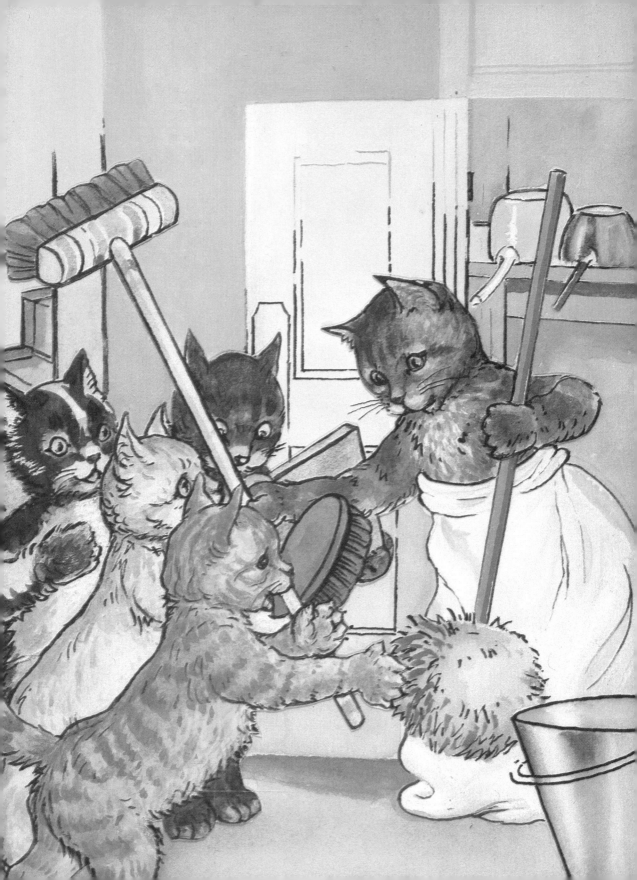

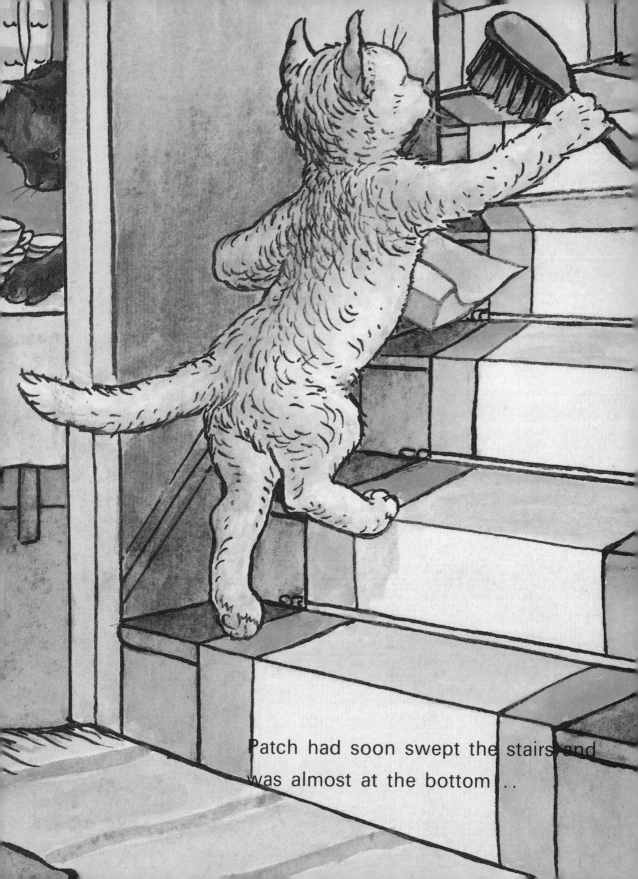

Patch had soon swept the stairs and was almost at the bottom . . .

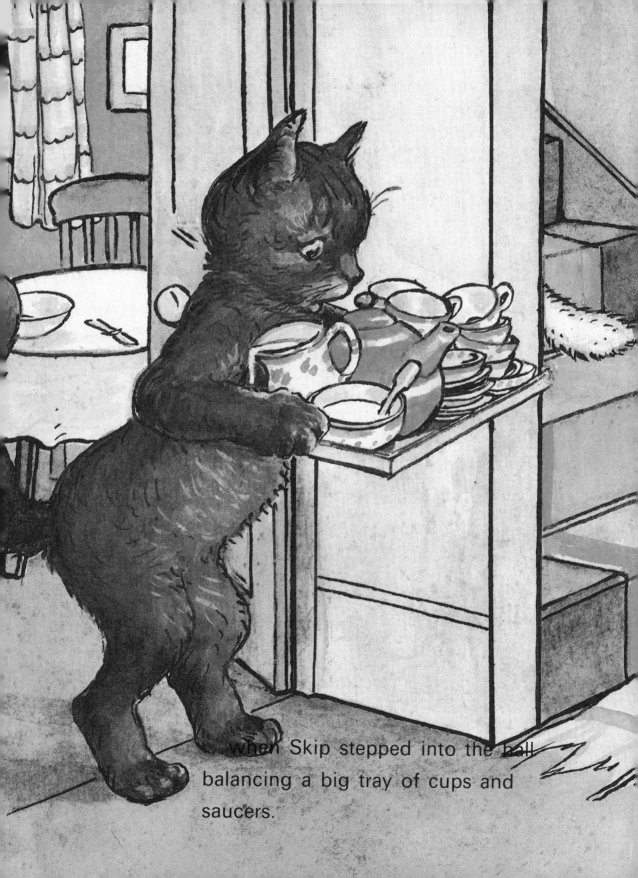

. . . when Skip stepped into the hall balancing a big tray of cups and saucers.

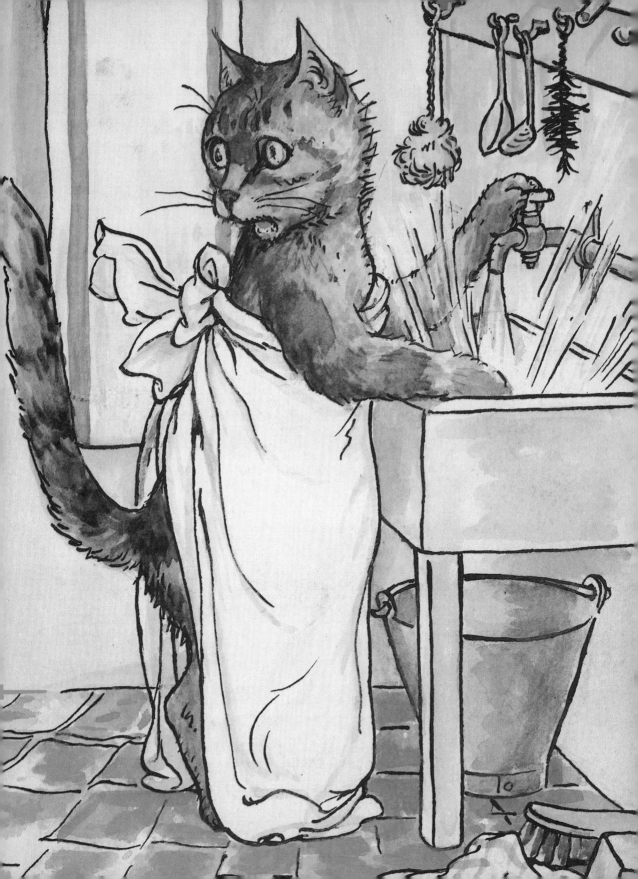

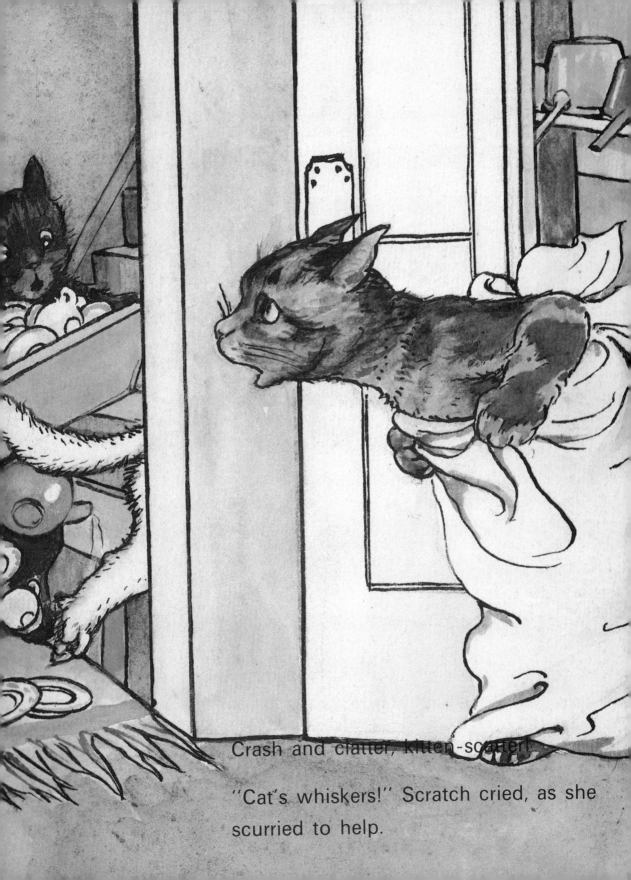

Crash and clatter, kitten-scatter!

"Cat's whiskers!" Scratch cried, as she
scurried to help.

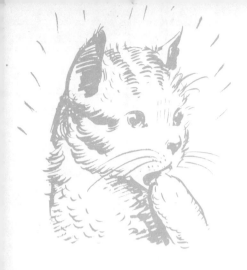

But Mama's apron was too long,
She flew right through the door.
Whoops!
Slipped and tripped, apron ripped,
Scratch joined them on the floor.

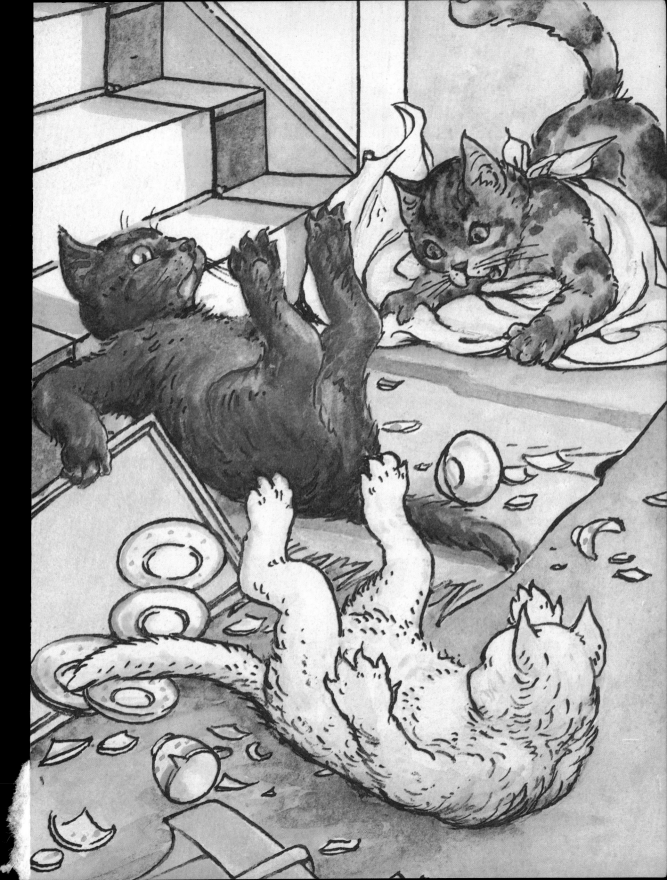

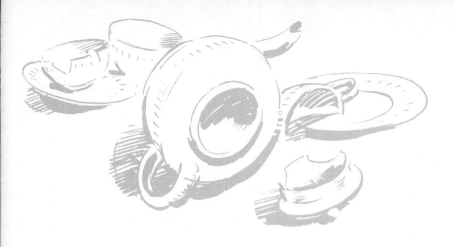

Shattered cups and crying kittens!

"We'll have to start again," sighed Scamp.

Scooter picked up Scratch and apron.

Patch and Skip picked up themselves.

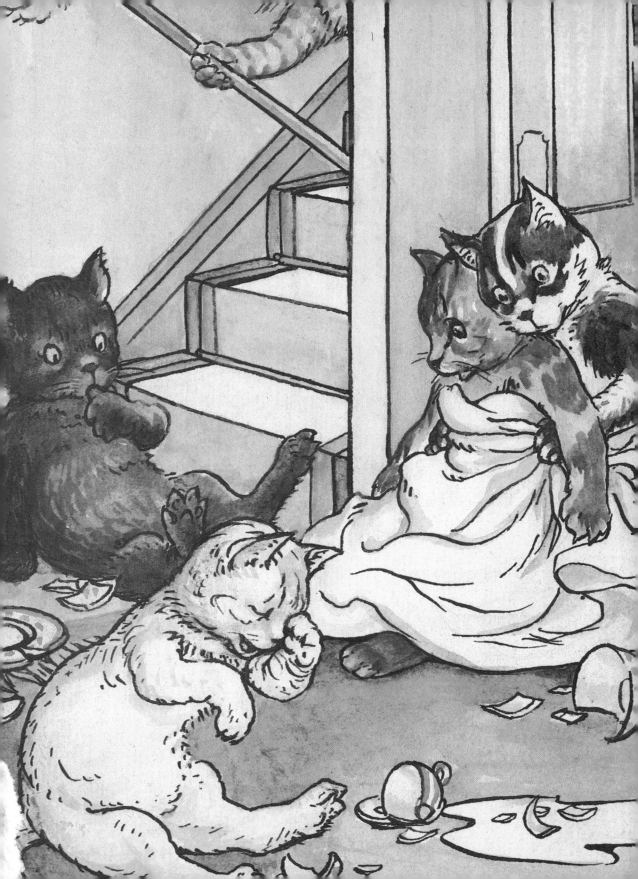

Soon cleaning up was almost fun again.

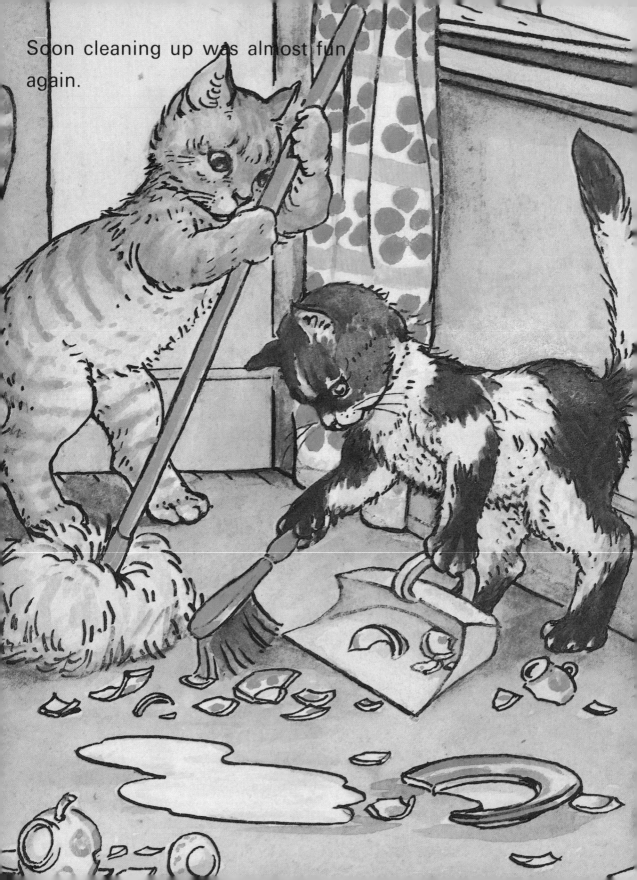

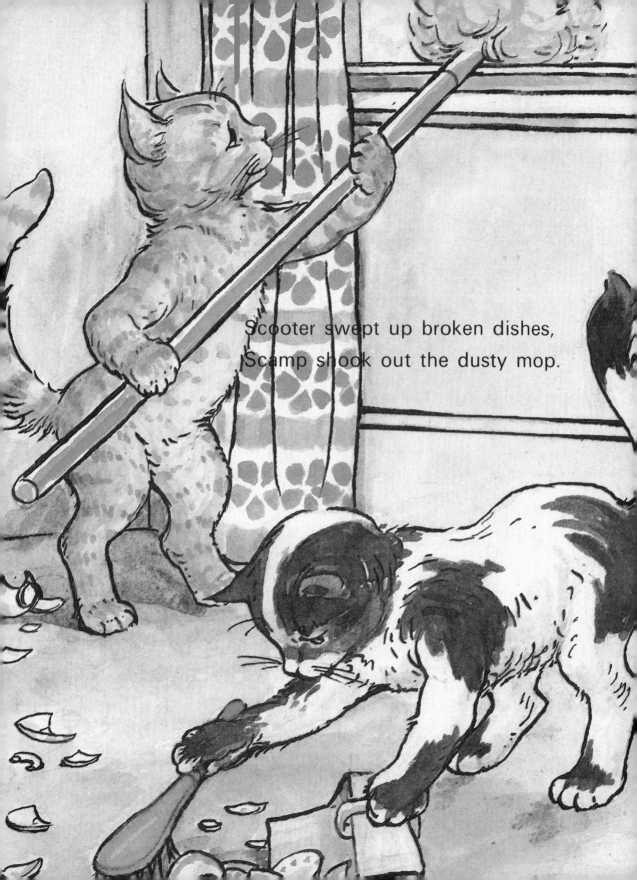

Scooter swept up broken dishes,
Scamp shook out the dusty mop.

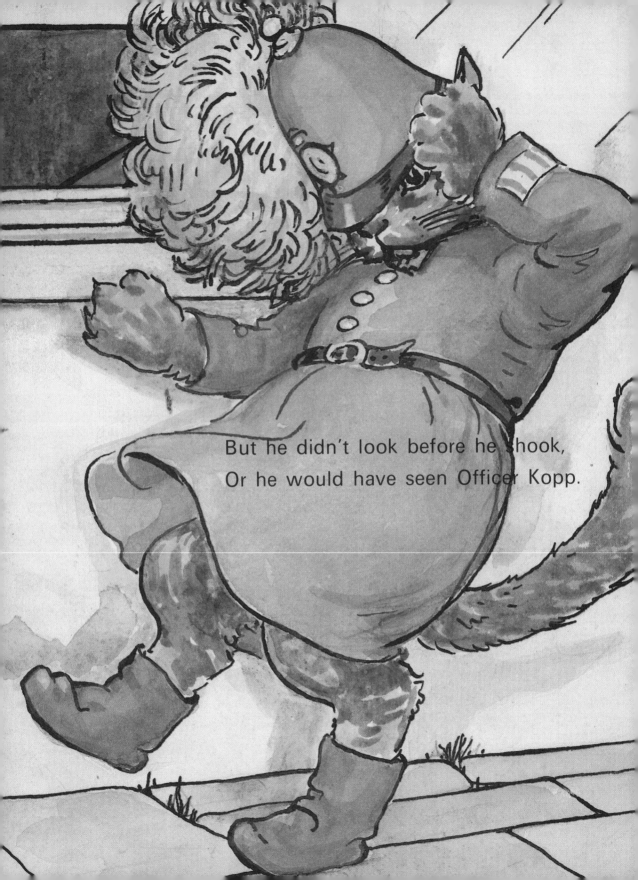

But he didn't look before he shook,
Or he would have seen Officer Kopp.

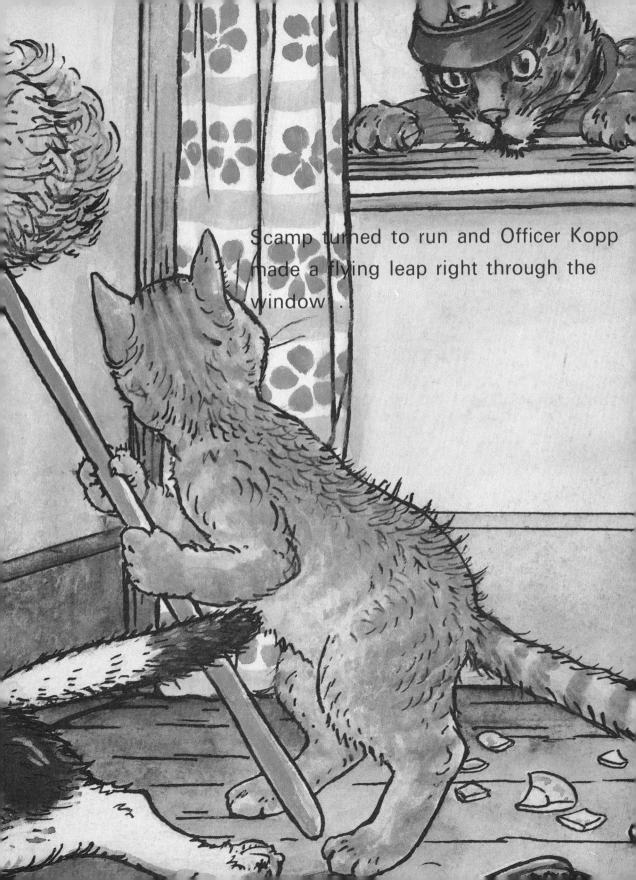

Scamp turned to run and Officer Kopp made a flying leap right through the window .

. . . just as Mama Cat returned home.

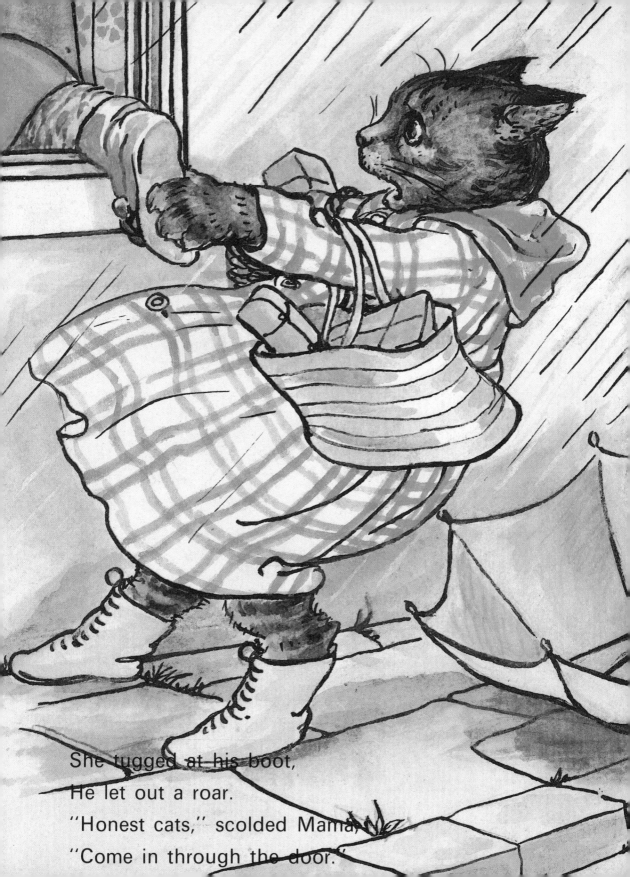

She tugged at his boot,
He let out a roar.
"Honest cats," scolded Mama,
"Come in through the door."

But what a surprise! It was Officer Kopp.
Said he, "I've been bopped on the head with a mop!"

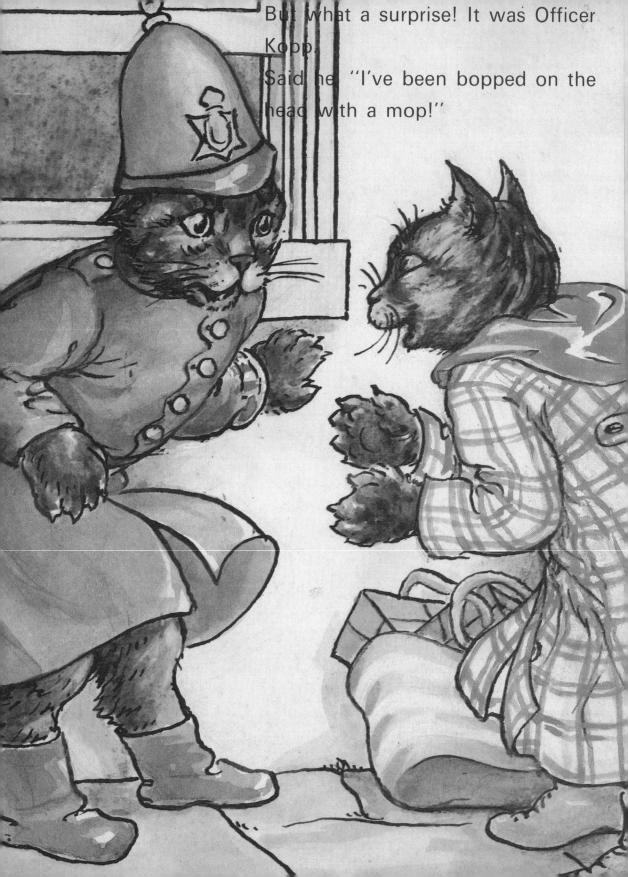

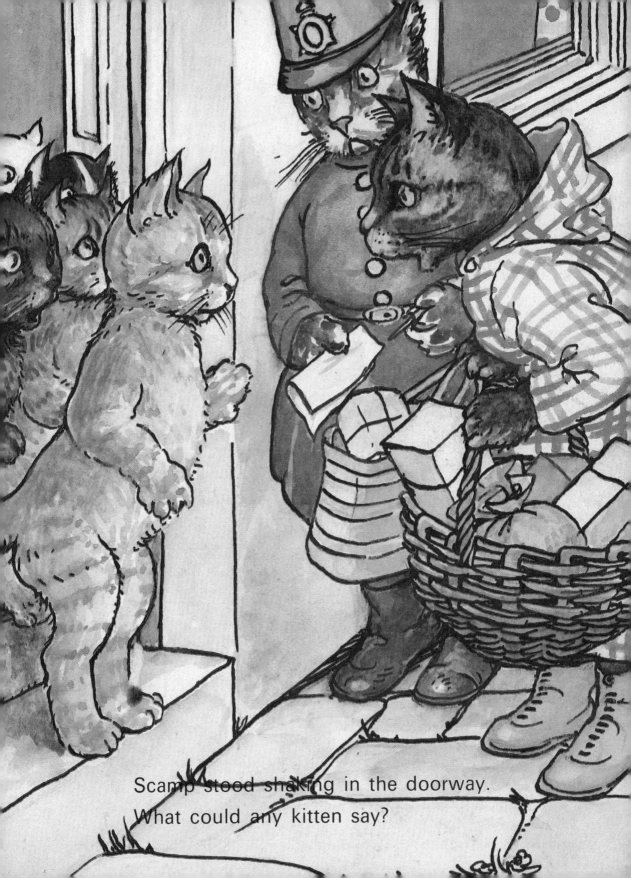

Scamp stood shaking in the doorway.
What could any kitten say?

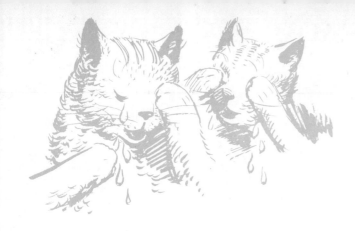

There was not a mew from Patch or
Scooter,
not a mew from Skip or Scratch.
Finally, sorry Scamp spoke up.
"We were helping with the cleaning.
didn't mean to hit your head."

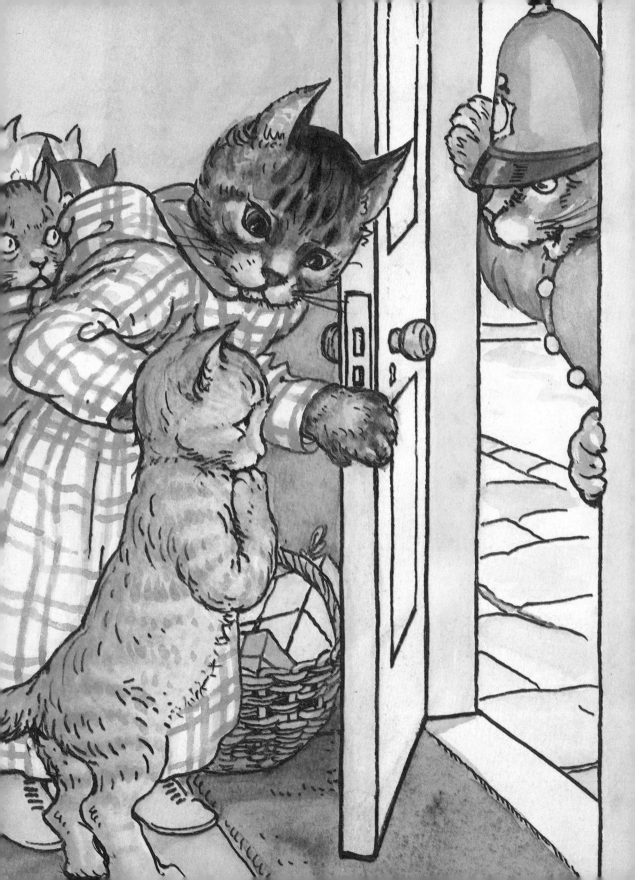

"Great catkins!" Mama shouted when she saw the shattered dishes. But she saw five sorry faces and her anger went away.

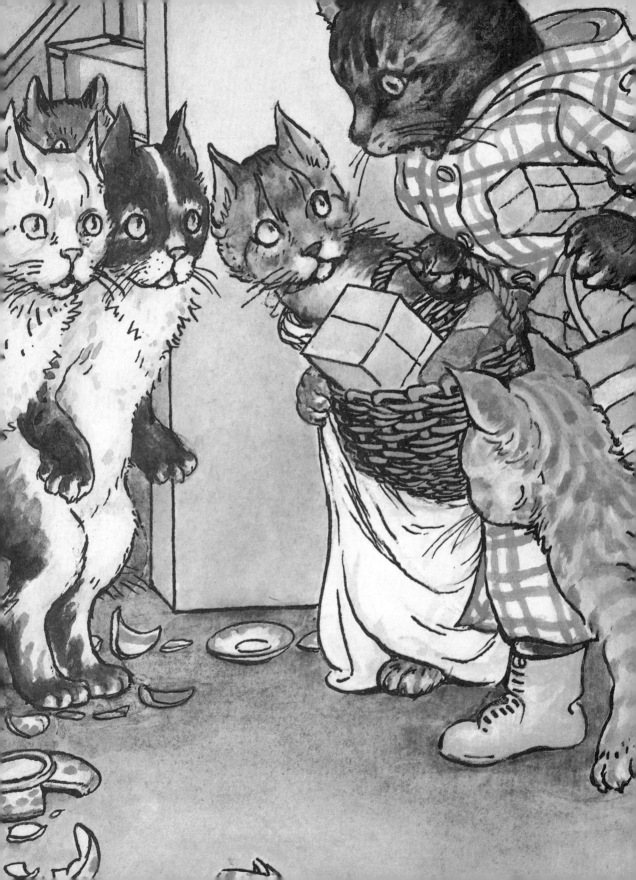

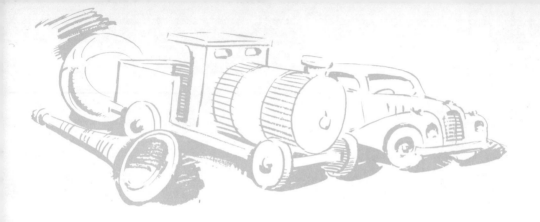

"Well, never mind," she said, "you tried
your best to help me."
Then she handed out the presents and
they all went off to play.
Scratch, Patch and Scooter, Skip and
Scamp had had a busy day.

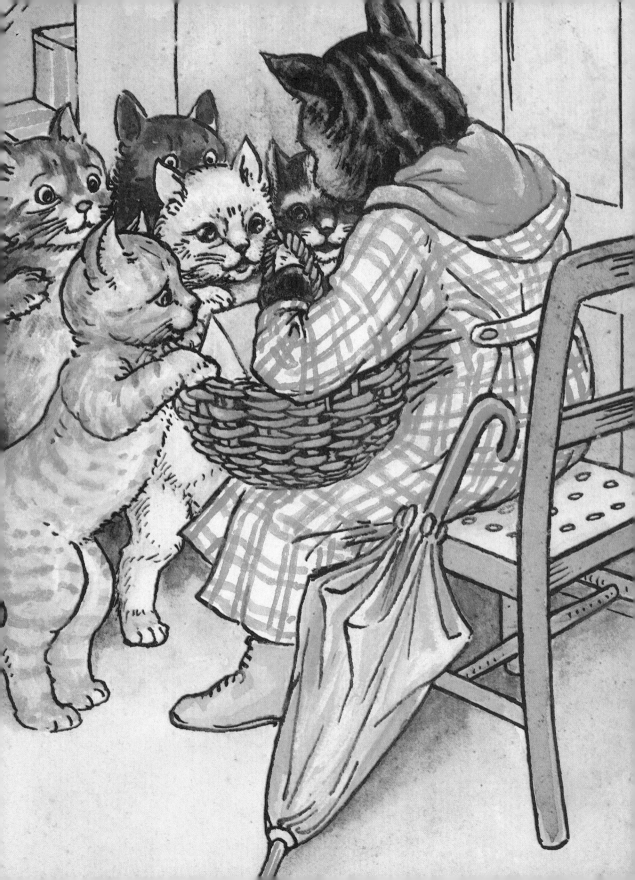

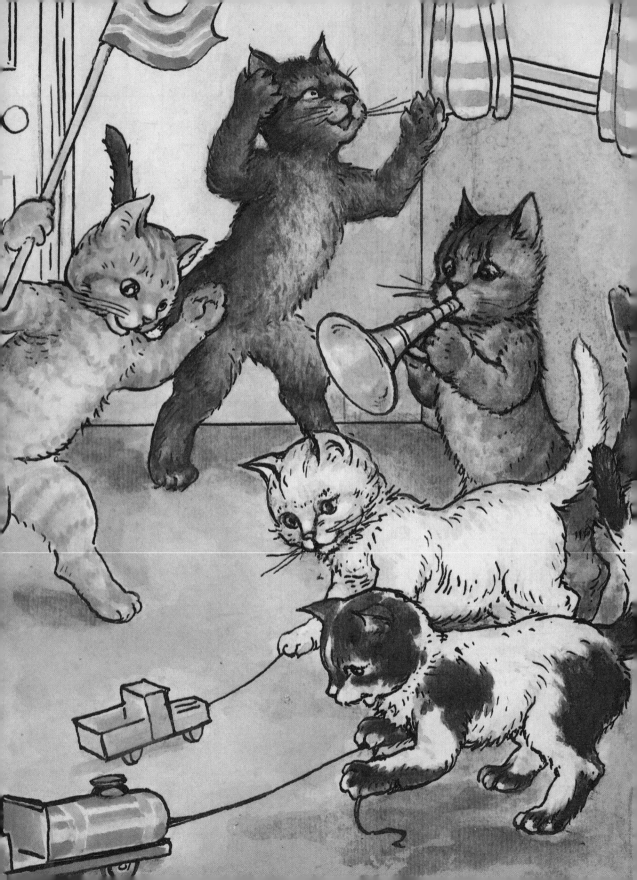